COUPLES THERAPY WORKBOOK

SEDUCTION AND STRATEGIES TO GET YOUR EX BACK

by Francesco Cibelli

Do you want to live happily in a relationship?

Do you want to make love flourish again after a period of crisis with your partner?

Do you want to save a marriage that seems compromised?

Do you want to win back your ex-partner after the breakup?

If the answer is yes, this is the right guide for you, for both men and women.

Francesco Cibelli, the author of the best seller "The secrets of the seducer: The playboy techniques," the most beloved and reviewed master in Italy in the field of seduction, after years of studies of the psychology of the couple, as well as field-tested techniques, has created this guide. It is useful for managing the couple's relationships, both in the physiological and pathological phase.

The first part is dedicated to providing strategies to make love grow in every phase of the relationship, from falling in love onwards. Emphasis is given to personal growth, the ontological difference between men and women, seduction even in an advanced phase of the couple and conflict management.

In the second part, the author teaches a step-by-step, almost surefire strategy to win back the partner after a breakup through techniques developed by the most famous psychologists on the subject that have been tested in the field.

Here the master of seduction will show us some success stories, personally experienced.

In this guide you will find:

How to live a dream couple relationship;

How to make love grow, in any state of the relationship;

How to apply the law of attraction and seduce your partner every day;

How to avoid fights;

How to deal with negative feelings;

How to deal with infidelity;

How to save the marriage before a breakup;

Mistakes to avoid when a relationship ends;

The No Contact Strategy;

Self-help techniques to overcome suffering and become more seductive;

Methods of reverse hypnotic seduction;

Strategies to win back the ex-partner;

Techniques to win back a partner after cheating;

How to manage the relationship after winning him/her back.

Here's what the readers say about this Guide:

"I was on the verge of breaking up my marriage and I didn't know what to do. I read this guide and rediscovered how to be seductive with my husband. Now we're happier than ever!"

Grazia Liorni

"My engagement was about to founder because of constant fighting and misunderstandings. After reading this guide, I understood how to manage conflicts and now everything is going well."

Andrea Sensi

"My ex-husband had left me for no apparent reason, and I was suffering. This book taught me a simple, but brilliant strategy to win him back. Thank you, Francesco Cibelli!"

Simona Longobardi

"I was desperate: my fiancée had cheated on me and wouldn't answer the phone anymore. "I wanted to win her back at all costs. With the method explained step by step in this guide, I first managed to regain contact and then I was able to prevail over my rival.

Forgiveness is a choice and the author will support us on this path!"

Carmine Soriente

Biography

Francesco Cibelli was born in Salerno in 1977. In 2003 he graduated with a degree in law and since 2004 he has been working as a civil servant. In 2006 he qualified to practice as a lawyer. He wrote the sylloge of poems Cuore Carminio, 2008, 0111 Edizioni; Lampi Fulgenti, 2018, sylloge of poems; The secrets of the seducer: The playboy techniques, 2018. He is quite active on social networks and, in particular, on Instagram and Facebook. He loves reading, nature and large groups of friends.

Summary

Introduction

Dear readers, after the extraordinary success of my book "The secrets of the seducer: The playboy techniques," I have been asked, by many of you, to continue my work with a guide on the management of couple relationships.

As I explained in that book, seduction is an art that can be learned: with the right strategies you can conquer any woman (or man).

The conquest can be the result of chance, a stroke of luck; in other cases, beautiful individuals or millionaires have no problem approaching the person they like; in other cases, the conquest can be caused by the classic "love at first sight."

The conquest phase may be induced by seduction strategies or may have natural and sometimes irrational origins.

Love, in fact, is not based on reason - or in any case not exclusively on rational elements - but on feelings and emotions: with reason alone, we will not be able to conquer any soulmate. It is necessary to make people fall in love, to be able to arouse emotions and magic: this is the wonder of love.

Being able to have a relationship with the person we like, therefore, can be the result of chance or the art of seduction.

Preserving and knowing how to manage the relationship is the product of an even finer art: it is not something you improvise! You have to take care of the relationship with the most important person in your life on a daily basis. And here too there are strategies to follow in order to live a happy and lasting relationship.

In my opinion, a happy life is based on the combination and balance of three pillars: health, self-fulfillment, and emotional relationships (friendship, cohabitation, marriage).

If one of these pillars were to be damaged, that person's life would be adversely affected. I believe that not even a millionaire can feel happy if he is alone in the world, not loved by anyone or with poor health. So, love, health and freedom to self-realize are the secrets of happiness.

Since one of the three pillars is the foundation of a happy life, it is essential to know how to manage and cultivate one's relationship as a couple.

Marriage, stable cohabitation, or engagement are the most exclusive and often the most important relationships in a person's life.

However, these love relationships are put to the test by elements both extrinsic and intrinsic to the couple.

On the one hand, the hectic life and stress to which we are subjected in today's society often affect relationships: there is no time to manage the relationship in the best possible way, which is in danger of deteriorating.

On the other hand, the couple themselves make the mistake of neglecting the love relationship: they tend to take everything for granted and end up making the daily routine prevail over the care of feelings.

These circumstances can make the couple unhappy. It is no coincidence that, according to the latest statistical research, divorce rates have increased at exponential levels in recent years, so much so that the legislature has also adapted to these changes by approving the laws on so-called "quick divorces."

Dear reader, this book has been written – and is addressed to both men and women – with the intention of helping you to optimize, strengthen, flourish, improve and brighten your love relationship. In addition, I have written the second part of the book with the aim of helping those who have suffered a breakup in their relationship to reconnect with their ex-partner, through virtually infallible techniques.

When you are in a happy and harmonious relationship, the serenity and love you feel is reflected in every other area of your life, making it much more harmonious, and free from stress.

And the happiness deriving from a satisfying sentimental situation allows you to increase your ability to concentrate, to work with more enthusiasm and to self-actualize yourself by bringing out your creative personality and your charisms. History also teaches us that brilliant minds, very often, have been supported by a loving and understanding partner.

I have written this guide, solicited by you, readers, on the basis of the numerous studies I have carried out on the subject of the psychology of the couple and especially the personal experiences I have lived through, in order to help you have a deeper understanding of the couple's relationship and marriage. In addition, I have personally developed effective strategies in order to win back the partner in the event of a breakup.

I feel I can help you, because besides being happily married for years and with children, I have lived through dozens of relationships, even lasting several years, and I have won back or had the chance to win back several exes. If you look at my previous work, "The secrets of the seducer: The playboy techniques," you will see that I am the most reviewed Italian author on the subject of seduction.

Therefore, whether you are in a relationship in the initial stage, engaged and planning to get married, already married or want to win back your ex-partner, I suggest you read this guide carefully because I am sure it will help you to make the most of the relationship with your soulmate and, more generally, to improve your life.

The four stages of love

According to psychologists and scholars of couples' relationships, love relationships go through four stages: infatuation, falling in love, disillusionment, and lasting love. In reality, many couples do not go through the third stage of the relationship, which is the most critical. Knowing these stages is important because, depending on the season in which the couple lives, it is possible to provide appropriate care so the love grows and does not wither.

Infatuation

This is the most beautiful stage of love: we feel happy and believe we have found the right person for us. We cannot even conceive of the idea of not loving our partner: we project all our dreams and desires onto them. We think that, after the disappointments of the past, our time has come to be happy and to have found eternal love. We value our partner's merits to the nth degree and completely set aside their faults.

There is a scientific explanation for all this: hormones such as serotonin, testosterone, estrogen, dopamine, and oxytocin affect our mind.

At this stage, it is very often that, in our mind, reality surpasses all hope and dreams: it is all wonderful.

In reality, the stage of infatuation can be the result of chance and there is no guarantee that you have found your soulmate. Sometimes, ideally unsuitable couples are formed rationally. This is because, in this stage, the emotional and unconscious element prevails. This stage can generally last from a single day (in the case of an obvious blunder) to eighteen months. Usually the couple passes this stage.

Falling in love

This is the stage in which the real couple is born: usually you go to live together, you are happy to share everything, you feel safe and pampered by your partner. Respect and esteem grow reciprocally, and you start to build, to make plans together: an individual thought is flanked by a "couple" thought.

In this amorous season there is no doubt that the initial enthusiasm will subside, leading to a more objective view of the couple. In any case, it is based on a more solid and rational bond: you continue to value the qualities of the other person and the defects are overcome by the right compromises. At this stage, the couple is happy and hopeful that this will last forever.

This cycle generally lasts until the seventh year and, being a positive stage for the couple, it is easy to reach the third cycle of love.

Disillusionment

Generally, after the seventh year of the couple's existence, we reach the negative stage of disillusionment: we realize the partner is a human being with their own strengths and weaknesses; we feel less loved and do not want to give the love that was given in the other stages of the relationship; past wounds re-emerge and affect the balance of the couple; we do not feel fulfilled and, in some cases, we feel chained to the partner.

This stage accentuates the tendency of men to shut themselves up in silence and appear detached;

at the same time, the tendency of women, at times, to be pessimistic and to see a dark and unhappy future is also accentuated.

This, unfortunately, is the stage in which many couples do not survive. There is not the will to work to build a solid and lasting love.

This is the stage in which both must struggle to understand the needs of the other person and ask for the help they need.

Love is a militia: you must build, be lovable day by day; this is the only way to build true love.

This guide is intended to help couples to overcome negative moments, to make feelings flourish again with the right strategies and to build a lasting love.

Lasting love

Not all couples will reach this stage, but for those that will, the benefits and satisfactions will be the highest: the partner is not the ideal savior we believed in the cycle of infatuation, but an ally who helped soothe the inner conflicts of the past, who loves us for who we are, with our virtues and flaws. The partner is a rock: the friend, the lover, the dearest person. Their support will never be lacking because they love us and know us deeply.

This is the stage in which you can have bliss and live intensely the love bond that was built with so much love. It is such a beautiful feeling you want to share it with others.

If two people have managed to build such a beautiful relationship, they want to project their happiness onto others, contributing to building a better world. The couple will leave a trail of light in the world.

The beginnings of a relationship

Let's assume you are in the early stages of a relationship. The first aspect to define is whether you want to commit yourself seriously to building something important with that person or not. Not everyone wants to build something serious and solid: sometimes you have other priorities, like career or fun; sometimes the other person is not ready.

Therefore, you have to try to understand if you and your partner are on the same wavelength and have the desire to build a solid and lasting relationship.

If the answer to the above question is yes, you need to define what key characteristics the partner must have to meet your expectations.

Then you need to know yourself: you need to understand your priorities, your values and the compromises you are willing to make; if these elements are clear to you, it will be easier for the person next to you to understand and respect them.

You then have to find out if you have the main life goals in common: love, work, sharing, and children.

You have to be aware that you will go through several difficulties and you have to be willing to overcome them with courage, tenacity and with the awareness that, once overcome, they will help to strengthen the relationship.

You should also consider that there are substantial differences between the life of a single person and the life of a couple; some are obvious, others are more subtle.

To live peacefully an engagement or a marriage, you need to review your habits, have the ability to adapt to the new status and be willing to accept the changes that have occurred.

If you have been single for many years, it is likely you will find it a little more difficult to adapt to change as you are used to your schedules, your habits, your hobbies, your friendships, without having to compromise with anyone. If you are a certain age and still live blissfully with your parents, adapting to change will require even more effort.

That does not mean you have to turn your pre-relationship life upside down. You have to remain consistent with your values; maintain some hobbies you care about; maintain your friendships.

This last element is fundamental: never neglect friendships. From personal experience, I can say that I have lived through dozens of relationships, even lasting ones: sometimes I ended the relationship; other times I was left. In all this, historical friendships have always been a fundamental point of reference in my life. In the most important moments of my existence, I have always had friends who have supported and cheered me up.

Therefore, it is necessary to change your habits, dedicating to the couple the time they deserve, but it is also necessary to carve out room for yourself.

As I mentioned above, the first step is to decide what kind of relationship you want to live in.

In this regard, the advice I want to give you is never to rush things: take the time to understand if that person is on your wavelength. One mistake many people make is to settle for and mate with the wrong person just out of loneliness or age. This is a huge mistake because a couple's relationship can be wonderful, but it can turn into the anteroom of hell, so it is better to be alone than live a destructive relationship.

Therefore, dismiss any decisions made based on emergency, fear and in a period of low self-esteem, and think that the right person for you will come at the right time and in unexpected ways and means.

If in a couple's relationship you find that there are often misunderstandings, incompatible character differences, completely different values, then stop and take your time.

If the relationship you are in does not satisfy you, psychologically traps you and does not make you happy, it is better to end it at the beginning, or before the wedding.

If you end a destructive relationship before it becomes too demanding, the pain and regret will be shorter and the breakup will involve fewer people; in the case of a more serious relationship, it will also affect families, mutual friendships and any children.

It is physiological that if you are trying to build a new, serious, and lasting relationship, you will have to face some difficulties. However, these small problems and difficulties will help you understand how willing you are to accept the other person. If your partner overreacts to small difficulties, and the slightest misunderstanding turns into a tragedy, then I advise you to end the relationship immediately.

I want to talk to you about an experience I had about ten years ago.

I was in a period of low self-esteem: I was no longer in my twenties and many family members were beginning to ask me why I was not engaged or married. So, I got engaged to a girl with a good job and a good reputation. Over time, however, I realized that she was too authoritarian: she wanted to decide for herself about our life; she wanted me to abandon my historical friendships; she even wanted me to change my values and my way of thinking.

I was not happy with her and, although in the eyes of the family we had what it takes to get married, I kept putting it off, year after year. Meanwhile, my grudge and resentment towards my partner increased. One day she gave me an ultimatum and asked me when I wanted to get married. With no hesitation, I answered her that I was never going to do it: it was a good decision!

If, on the other hand, you feel that the relationship completely satisfies you, makes you happy and fulfilled, that you get along well, have similar tastes and personalities, then follow your emotional side and without fear build something important! A few months are enough to understand if she or he is the right person.

With my authoritarian ex-girlfriend, I hesitated for years to build something important because we were not on the same wavelength.

However, when I met my wife, I immediately understood that she was my soulmate: she is a beautiful Belarusian, sweet and understanding, we have the same values and goals. I am happy with her. I will not hide the fact that we got married after only seeing each other three times. It was, for my part, the wisest decision of my life! Now, when I wake up in the morning, I often contemplate the blond angel next to me, our sweet children and the day starts with a radiant smile.

The second step, as I mentioned above, is to know yourself. This important aspect should not be underestimated: it is essential that you not only know your virtues and qualities, but also your flaws and any limits that block you. Only in this way, can you begin a path of personal growth, so you can overcome these limits and improve both individually and within the couple.

When you really learn to know yourself, you can express who you are with more confidence and freedom and this will allow your partner to accept you as you really are.

Many people try to appear in a different way than they really are, and this is not good for the relationship because the very essence of the relationship cannot be considered authentic.

Seduction strategies – sometimes including lies or tricks – can only serve in the approach phase to stimulate the emotional side of the future partner. However, if you want to build the relationship on a solid and lasting basis you have to be sincere and authentic. To do this, you first need to get to know each other.

I advise that you learn to observe the other person with curiosity and interest, to ask specific questions and to listen carefully to their answers. In this way, you can penetrate the personality of your loved one. Some people, mistakenly, concentrate on talking without properly listening to their partner. However, keep in mind that when you talk, you say things you already know, while it is when you listen that you can discover and understand new things and the relationship can be strengthened.

The third step is to understand if you share common goals: the will to live together, to love each other, to respect each other, to share the same values. To understand this, you need to take time to understand and get to know each other.

If you notice right from the start of a relationship that there is no sense of protection, if there is no genuine love, if you see that the other person is not completely present, or is only partially interested in things that concern you, do not expect that these things will change with the passage of time.

On the contrary, as we have already seen, over time these failings may even increase. The enthusiasm on the part of the other person, the sense of happiness is fundamental and must be present in the first encounters.

The factors underlying a happy and satisfying relationship are few, but they are essential: their absence indicates the other person is probably not ready to commit himself or herself completely or that he or she does not intend to engage in a serious and lasting relationship. In this case, the relationship should be ended without delay.

How to make love grow

Once the prerequisites are in place for the couple to have a future, it is necessary to define what ingredients are useful for the growth and consolidation of love.

Some of these elements are: being lovable, being mutually responsible, caring for each other, communicating, taking time, being sincere and being transparent.

If you are not aware of any necessary elements to make a relationship work, sooner or later – and certainly once past the initial enthusiasm – the relationship itself will be compromised and you may feel lost in the complexities of life as a couple.

It is particularly useful in a conjugal relationship, or in a couple's relationship in general, to care for each other and ensure the relationship grows harmoniously and peacefully.

First, you have to be lovable if you want to be loved. The harshness and the fights move the hate and that's why many couples break up. No one has forced you to stay in the same bed or live unhappily. So you must try to shine with virtue and be cheerful. The partner must rejoice in your presence. As a couple, you should live better than when you were single. This seems a trivial element, but it is essential to life as a couple. So avoid systematic quarrels!

Secondly, responsibility is a key point in a couple's relationship and, for there to be balance, it must be mutual. Both partners are equally responsible for the relationship itself and its development. Potentially, we might have a chance to argue every day, but it is necessary to be responsible: always look beyond the surface of appearances and wonder what is behind the behavior.

Please note that, as we shall also see later on, men and women speak, in part, different languages, and misunderstandings can often arise. If, for instance, the woman says, "This house is always messy!", the man might understand it as, "It's your fault if the house is always messy: you never do anything and I don't want to be with such a man."

However, knowing the female psyche, it is more likely that the woman is saying, "Today I am tired, and the house is in a mess. Would you give me a hand?"

Only by being responsible can you can solve every problem and misunderstanding: you must be open and not critical towards your partner.

Thirdly, you must take care of each other. The first step to doing this is to love yourself. Once you have learned to love yourself you can share your love with your partner and other people.

Until you have learned to love yourself, and so as long as you look for love on the outside rather than on the inside, you will always be insecure and transmit this insecurity through your behavior.

You cannot give what you do not have. That is why you must love yourself, and develop the love inside you, to be able to give it to your partner. If you love yourself, you are a loving person, you behave lovingly, and thus automatically become a person to love.

There are small daily gestures that show care for another person and, in the long run, to strengthen the relationship. Short words like "thank you," "sorry," or "please" do not cost anything, but they are a powerful tool to show your care and appreciation.

You should never take things for granted and you should never neglect the small daily attentions: you will thus avoid many quarrels and misunderstandings.

Treat the other person with respect and love so they do not feel neglected and the other person will do the same to you. Show gratitude for having someone you love and who loves you by your side. Be thankful for whatever gift your partner gives you and you will see the gifts of love will increase.

Fourth, being able to communicate is another essential factor in a relationship: the absence of communication can cause a relationship to deteriorate over time.

In this regard, I would like to remind you that when you are thinking, no one listens to you and you cannot expect another person to guess what you are thinking or what you would like. As much as you can achieve a certain degree of intimacy, no partner can read your mind as St. Pio could. If you have something to say, positive or negative, say it loud and clear without allusions or other similar games.

Dialogue is essential for a successful relationship. If you see that your partner is worried about something, be caring and understanding.

In particular, the woman needs to share her problems more than the man. This does not necessarily mean having to find a solution to the problems or change the situation. Many times, it is enough for a man to listen with love and understanding to make his partner feel better.

When it comes to communication, one mistake to avoid is taking things for granted: love must be cultivated every day, otherwise it withers. Therefore, often remind the other person that you love them, that it is important to you and that their benefit and well-being are essential to you.

When there are problems, talk about them with your partner: in the long run, stifled emotions accumulate until they explode and cause serious quarrels in the relationship. This advice should be borne in mind especially for economic problems that many people tend not to want to deal with. These are resolved through dialogue, compromise, mutual responsibility, and love.

Fifth, time for the partner is an essential element. If you think carefully, you will agree with me that time is the most precious gift we can give a person. Time is even more important than money: not even millionaires can buy time.

Therefore, do not make the mistake of devoting a lot of time to the initial phase of the relationship and then neglecting the partner in the other phases of the relationship.

Think of a couple's relationship as a plant: it should be cared for every day, no matter how old it is. The same goes for a couple's relationship: it takes care and dedication, enthusiasm, positivity, the desire to discover new things together, to have common goals and dreams to achieve.

Obviously, the time to devote to the partner must be profitable: if you have to communicate with your partner only to complain or quarrel, that is not quality time. Nobody likes to spend time with a complaining, critical and pessimistic person and your partner is no exception!

Many spouses or cohabitants often stop communicating under the pretext of lack of time, hard work or commitments.

In the frenzy of everyday life, you might easily neglect your relationship which, on the contrary, should be among your priorities. Remember that love is one of the pillars of a happy life.

Never neglect love. If, for instance, you are a doctor and you have ten patients a day who leave you no room for your partner, immediately reduce the number of patients to nine. Make your partner your tenth patient. The most important patient.

Sixth, trust and transparency are also powerful weapons to strengthen love.

If you develop love and self-confidence first, you will then be so confident that you will face the world with your head held high and without fear.

If you love yourself, you will not adopt attitudes and behaviors that could harm you or other people: as a result, you will always make choices that show esteem and respect for yourself and others; you will not tell lies and others will tend not to do so with you; you will have no problem acting and expressing yourself in total honesty and others will be inclined to do the same with you.

Therefore, if you treat your soulmate with trust and honesty, your partner will do the same to you. If you tell lies, criticize, and treat your partner with little respect, expect to receive the same treatment.

These six tips, intended to strengthen the life of the couple, may seem trivial. But consider that only a few can apply them. So, try to cultivate and improve your relationship day by day, and you will see that as time goes by, you will be increasingly happy both inside and outside the couple.

The law of attraction

We have so far dealt with the preconditions for strengthening a couple's relationship from a rational point of view. The rules set out in the previous chapter succeed, if applied, in bringing a love relationship into a comfort zone: you can count unconditionally on the other person, you share important values, you have trust and respect towards your partner.

However, as important as it may be, being able to arrive in a comfort zone only represents 50% of the path you must take to arrive at a happy relationship: it only covers the rational aspect.

However, love also feeds on irrational and emotional aspects. Once we are sure that we are loved by the other person, we tend by nature to take everything for granted and to care less about the relationship.

It sounds crazy, but we are as instinctive as children. Imagine a child longing for a toy. He cries and despairs, even for days, until, once obtained, he receives momentary satisfaction and plays with that toy for a few days. Often, however, we find that already after two weeks, that child will no longer play with the toy he has so longed for and will be attracted to another toy he does not have.

What does the example of the child teach us? That as long as there is a lack of a thing or a person, there will be attraction for that thing or that person: there will be a spasmodic desire for that thing or that person and this desire will push us like a magnet towards the object of our desire.

Therefore, the premise of the attraction is lack, scarcity. Lack, scarcity attract. Even in business, if you think about it, the more there is scarcity, the more there will be attraction and that thing will be precious.

In a couple's relationship, the law of attraction is fully applicable and is worth 50% of the path that leads to the happiness of the relationship itself.

If one of the partners is too present and available within the couple, it will certainly not appear attractive and will lead the other partner to feel too confident in the relationship and stop giving.

In other cases, the overly loved partner may even feel precious and believe that everything is due to him or her. In other cases, the overvalued partner might feel besieged and tend to reject the other person. There are so many cases of divorce on the grounds – or excuse – that the partner was too obsessive, too jealous!

Couples' relationships are certainly 50% based on rational comfort: kindness, romanticism, sincerity, common goals; but another 50% is based on attraction, mystery, the emotional and primordial side of man.

Seduction must not be relegated only to an initial phase of the relationship but must be permanent: we must court the other person forever. No one is bound to you: love is built day by day and there will never be a point of arrival. Love must always be enriched with new stimuli.

I remember that when I was a boy, I was attracted to pretty girls who were often out of my league.

I was not attracted at all by the good girls of the Franciscan youth, a Catholic association that I frequented at the time: they may have been nice, family lovers, sincere and rich in values, but they did not attract me.

On the contrary, I was attracted by pretty, flashy girls, desired by many, with many relationships behind them. When I was able to be with one of them, I committed myself to giving my best: I thought I was lucky because among many suitors they had chosen me; I did everything not to be betrayed. I was like a magnet. And my magnet did not go to the good girls, but to the flashy and apparently unreachable ones.

Dear female Reader, how many times has it happened to you, too, not to be attracted to a good guy, but to one who wasn't exactly a "saint"? The answer lies in the law of attraction: we are attracted by scarcity, by what we might not have, by what is mysterious.

Sometimes you just like what is nasty. There are pathological cases whereby certain girls (or boys) are attracted to taken or married people. In most cases they will suffer, but afterwards they will not look for a good single guy, but yet another a complicated relationship.

The science of relationships is complex, but with the study of behaviors, it is possible to develop strategies that can help to create happy couple relationships, which reconcile both the need for comfort and the need for attraction.

Therefore, I advise you to take short periods of time away from your partner: sometimes they must miss you. At the same time take care of your image, try to be a successful person; in this way you will attract not only others, but also your own partner, in a continuous game of seduction.

Sometimes you may lead your partner to believe you have admirers. This could rekindle a passion that has been dormant for some time within the couple. Obviously, you have to be moderate and live the whole thing as a game. One must never exaggerate and create arguments.

You will have heard many times that in love, the winner is the one who flees. Actually, in a couple's relationship, that's exactly how things are. According to the law of attraction, if you distance yourself for a few days, you will induce your partner to miss you and thus attract him or her.

Once you are back, the desire to be together will be enormous. It is as if your partner comes back to you with an immense thirst; all you have to do is water him or her.

Dear reader, I want to give you one last piece of advice. You must only leave for a few days and at a time when there is no particular disagreement with your partner. An absence that is too long may cause the partner to miss you less and less and to establish new acquaintances. I do not think this is one of your goals!

The management of marriage or co-habitation

Back now to a rational approach, we will discuss the main factors leading to a stable, solid, and lasting marriage or cohabitation.

In this regard there are some simple but highly effective rules to follow: help each other; keep the romantic aspect of the relationship alive; try to make economic progress.

Living together is not always easy, especially because everyone has their own habits, preferences, desires, and everyone has their own background which necessarily differs from that of their partner.

To prevent misunderstandings and conflicts from arising, it is necessary to lay down certain rules or customs to be observed. It is necessary to establish which situations or values neither of the two is willing to compromise on. In this respect, we must be sincere and clear in expressing our needs. Once this is done, these rules must be respected at any cost by both partners.

Mutual help

Both partners in a couple's relationship must deal with certain responsibilities and commitments. This is essential for the balance and serenity of family life. It is fair that everyone has their own workload, in order not to burden the other person and make the relationship work harmoniously.

These tasks and responsibilities must be agreed, case by case, and vary from couple to couple according to each person's inclinations and the compromises that have been reached.

It is essential to share tasks and responsibilities in a balanced way. If one of the partners were overburdened by family commitments in a disproportionate way, it would certainly bring out, over time, resentment, and other negative feelings for the survival of the couple.

Sharing tasks and family commitments is not only fair, but it is rewarding, because you feel you are the protagonist of the creation of a harmonious and happy family.

It is also important not only to help each other, but to learn how to properly ask your partner for the help you need. It is essential to ask for help in a straightforward manner. And this is difficult for both men and women.

However, men, by their very nature, tend to ask for the help they need directly.

Women, on the other hand, ontologically find it more difficult to ask for help and, even more so, to ask for direct help.

The woman, when in love, is naturally inclined to give herself totally to her partner to make him happy: she offers love and help without being asked for it. The woman somehow tries to prevent her partner's requests by offering help and support in a thousand different ways. Even when she finds that she is not adequately reciprocated, she continues to give without asking, in the hope that sooner or later the man will reciprocate.

Unfortunately, however, the man is less inclined than the woman to give, to self-give without being asked. Indeed, a man who is not asked for help will be led to believe that he already gives enough to his partner.

This situation will, in many cases, lead the woman to resentment and, the moment she decides to ask her partner for help, her requests will appear as a demand in the eyes of the other. And I can assure you that men do not like demands: demands often lead to conflict.

One mistake women often make is to ask for help indirectly. This way of asking generates conflict, because the man cannot always understand what is behind an indirect request.

Let us take an example. If a woman is tired and does not feel like making lunch, she could say to her partner, "I don't have time to make lunch today." This is the classic example of an indirect request that upsets the man. In fact, the latter translates: "I've been working too hard and I'm tired: it's your duty to take me out to lunch."

I advise women to ask directly. In the example above, the correct way to ask is as follows: "Can we have lunch out today?"

This direct request is generally well received by the man because there is no resentment and it is an invitation to do something different together.

Other indirect expressions that may irritate men are to use can or could in the formulation of requests. It is preferable not to ask, "Could you take me to lunch?" as this is an indirect request. Better to ask, "Honey, will you take me to lunch?"

Keeping the passion and romantic side of the relationship alive

The best relationship is achieved when your partner can be considered both your best friend and your lover.

Friendship is a noble feeling that involves dialogue, trust, sharing values; being lovers involves passion, mutual attraction both mental and carnal.

Romanticism is certainly an important element to cultivate in long-term relationships: it can be compared to a rose bush in which there is cyclical flowering.

A woman could awaken her husband's romanticism by always showing up well-dressed and well-groomed even at home and never appearing neglected.

A man could awaken the romance of his soul mate by making her feel important, loved and appreciated, giving her frequent compliments, unexpected gifts and taking her out to dinner in a particular restaurant.

It is also necessary to cultivate the passionate and emotional aspect of the couple.

While it is true that passion may diminish over time in a natural process that happens in all relationships, it is also true, however, that there are seductive strategies that serve to rekindle passion.

Never take anything for granted. The partner is still a person with feelings, needs and emotions: one must not fall into apathy and boredom, but rather discover new treasures every day and give oneself to each other in a different way.

It is essential to revive the fire of passion often with new stimuli, to alienate oneself for short periods of time and then to win back with greater ardor.

The sexual aspect is also fundamental in a relationship. Even if many years have passed, it is necessary, with imagination, to look for new facets of pleasure: the woman, for instance, might invent artifices to make herself desired; the man might instead learn techniques to postpone the extreme bliss and fully satisfy the woman.

Economic stability

One of the pillars of a happy life is also economic independence or financial stability. Money is often a source of stress and arguments even in relationships.

If trust, sincerity, and transparency are the basis of the relationship, there will be no reason to hide anything on the subject of money as well.

Face any difficulty with the confidence that together with your partner everything can be solved. You have to share everything, even economic problems.

If you want to hide financial problems from your partner, you risk feeling subjugated and your consequent lack of serenity will be reflected in your behavior, causing misunderstandings and arguments within your relationship.

In order to live more peacefully, depending on the availability of funds, it is preferable to establish rules together, draw up a revenue and expenditure plan and define a budget for your needs, weekly or monthly.

The more accurate you are in drawing up this sort of family balance sheet, the more smoothly everything will flow.

Part of the economic revenue should also be saved to cope with periods of emergency. It is also advisable to try to increase the income, if possible, without neglecting the time to devote to the couple.

The rules of harmony

Now I want to tell you some secrets that will help you to blend differences and create harmony in your relationship or in your marriage.

To achieve the happiness and harmony you seek in couple's life you need to be open to change and willing to compromise.

Compromising, however, does not mean stifling your needs or your point of view. Compromising means, above all, looking for the positive aspect of the partner in every situation; it means stopping highlighting the mistakes and defects of the other person and emphasizing their virtues and qualities.

Compromising therefore means tolerating the partner's flaws and habits that you do not share and appreciating, on the contrary, what good and beautiful things they have to offer you; it means evaluating the other person from a general point of view, without highlighting the flaws.

Avoid reprimanding your partner about behavior or habits that you do not like, unless they are of particular importance to you.

If you argue with the other person every day, make remarks often, or emphasize every little thing, you will lose credibility and be seen as a grumpy person.

If you are used to complaining about everything, your partner will not listen to you when a situation disturbs you in a particular way.

If, on the other hand, in most situations, you live the relationship in a proactive and harmonious way, when you have something important to say, your partner will be inclined to listen to you carefully.

The same situation occurs in parent-children relationships. If parents constantly scold their children, they get used to this type of behavior and no longer pay attention to it.

Another suggestion I want to give you is not to upset your partner with phrases like "I told you so!" or "I was right!". These attitudes create antagonisms within the couple and are by no means an added value. In some cases, they are perceived by the partner as ridiculous behavior.

When I said these negative phrases, I was often told, "You sound just like an old wise man!"

You must aim to create a loving and serene environment in your home and to instill harmony in every situation and in every relationship.

Score points with your partner

There are useful attitudes to gain points with the partner.

Women and men, being physiologically different, attribute points differently.

Women need to be loved and supported with many small positive things that a partner can do. Only by doing many little things will a man make his woman feel loved and valued.

It is not appropriate on the part of man to perform striking actions (e.g. gifting a new car), if he then neglects the little things he did at the beginning of the relationship. For the woman, the time you can devote to your family is more important than the extra money you can earn by working harder.

Here are some examples of positive behaviors that men could adopt in order to gain points towards their soulmate: offering practical help when she is tired; listening to her without distractions when she is vulnerable; often saying "I love you" to her; making little surprises (bringing flowers or sweets); writing a little poem; planning little romantic getaways.

Man, on the other hand, is inclined to award points to his soulmate when he is lovingly appreciated and not judged.

Here are some examples of what women can do to make a man happy: not punishing a man when he makes a mistake; asking for support without being demanding; sincerely appreciating moments of intimacy; welcoming a man with love after a period of separation; not giving advice on how to do something better (such as driving or fixing something at home).

Knowing how to score points with your partner is fundamental in order to optimize the energies that lead to the harmony of the relationship.

Take a positive and active attitude

Taking a constructive and pragmatic daily attitude is fundamental for your well-being and the well-being of your life as a couple.

This attitude must exist both when family relationships are positive and in the event of difficulties and disputes between spouses or partners.

Be pragmatic: it is better to live in harmony than to be on the side of reason. What is the point of being right if you live within an unhappy couple?

So, you have to practice finding the right compromises: you have to accept the flaws of the partner and the different points of view. One cannot control the other's mind. What you can do is express your points of view with love and listen carefully to the other person's needs. The feeling of love, the emotions, help to merge the couple into one family entity better than a treatise on reason!

Unconditional love leads you to happiness

Love always wins; it is the answer to every problem. With a loving attitude towards yourself, towards the people in your life and towards your soulmate, there is nothing you cannot solve.

The path to love is understanding, which allows one to go beyond forgiveness and develop compassion and empathy.

It is not appropriate to judge a person's behavior: you have to try to put yourself in their shoes and understand what is at the origin of a behavior.

Forgiving does not mean justifying behavior that you do not approve of; it means understanding the other person's reasons and moving on without accusing them.

Once that is done, you'll decide how to behave according to the specific situation. The important thing is, before reacting, to stop and think about what is at the origin of a certain behavior.

Such an attitude together with unconditional love and appreciation for yourself, for the people in your life and for your partner allow you to achieve the happiness you desire.

Happiness, contrary to what one might think, does not depend on external circumstances, but is intrinsic to a person's spirit. To be happy, you must develop appreciation and gratitude for all the people or things that life offers you.

Be the change you want to see in the other person

You cannot authoritatively change another person. You cannot pretend to change a person, but you have to accept them for who they are. The only way you can help a person to change, to improve, is through your example, through your actions. It is the results you achieve, in every area of life, that can influence people to follow a certain virtuous behavior. Words are of little use.

Each individual is different: they have their own opinions, experiences and unique characteristics. You cannot expect another person to share your opinion or decide to do what you think is right.

If you want to see a change, change yourself first: you are the only person over whom you have total control.

When you do that, you will see that your partner will change in turn, when they want to, and when they're ready to.

Take care of your personal growth

It is not the external conditions that must change for you to get results and improve your life: the change must start with you. In fact, external conditions are a reflection of your way of thinking and therefore of your way of acting and relating to life.

Working on personal growth will help you make changes and improvements in every area of your life, including your relationship or marriage.

I suggest you read books, listen to audio and follow personal growth programs to understand how your mind works and what is the connection between what you think, your beliefs, your reality and the experiences you live. Only then can you understand how you approach the world and how the world reacts to the image you offer of yourself;

only then can you consciously create your happy life.

Through personal growth programs, you will be more likely to succeed in both the personal and work spheres. And successful people are certainly more seductive, even within a couple's relationship.

Ontological differences between men and women

In order to make a couple relationship work at its best, it is always necessary to keep in mind that men and women are ontologically different: they have different characteristics, values and perceptions of reality.

One of the reasons behind fights and misunderstandings within the couple is that men often forget to communicate with women, treating them like men; at the same time, women forget to deal with men, treating them like a female friend.

They forget one fundamental element: men and women speak completely different languages.

By their nature, men love career, power, goals, and achievements. They are more interested in technological objects that can be useful to their work success than in people. They are not lovers of psychology and romance novels: while women dream of a romantic love story, men dream of having a car as powerful as a Ferrari.

For men to feel fulfilled, solving problems alone is of paramount importance. For these reasons, men hate it when women try to correct them, to improve them with unsolicited advice: for them, such interference consists in a lack of confidence in their own abilities.

The tendency of men to be pragmatic is also reflected in their communication with women: if they open up and talk about their upsets, the man will immediately try to find a solution to the problem; however, he does not understand that, often, the woman does not want to have a solution to the problem, but only to be listened to, understood, pampered.

Women, on the other hand, by nature give more value to feelings, interpersonal relationships, communication, emotions. They are more intuitive and instinctive; this is also reflected in the way they dress: depending on their mood they can change clothes several times a day.

They love psychology and personal growth. They are also very intuitive: they can anticipate the moods of their interlocutors by understanding what they need; they are inclined to offer help, even if they are not asked for it.

However, offering assistance to a man can often give him the feeling that he is incompetent to solve problems in a woman's eyes and feel humiliated. While the woman has no problem expressing her feelings, even negative ones, the man is more introverted about his moods.

Therefore, to reach a man, the woman should show confidence in his abilities, admire him, without wanting at all costs to improve anything of his work.

At the same time, in order to reach a woman, a man should listen to her attentively, interpenetrating in her state of mind, without offering a solution, but indulging her, making her feel loved and valued with small gestures and attention.

Another fundamental difference between men and women lies in stress management.

When a man has a problem, he closes in on himself and doesn't want to talk about it with anyone, neither with his woman, nor with friends or family: he needs a few hours or a few days to analyze the problem in all its facets and then solve it. If he cannot solve the problem, he seeks some distraction by continuing in his state of passivity. Only after solving his difficulties will he become receptive again.

All men, periodically, close in on themselves to face certain problems: it is their nature.

This attitude of the man can often be a reason for conflict with the woman, as the latter suddenly sees herself neglected, excluded, and may believe that she is not loved and considered enough by the man.

In these moments, the woman tends to get closer to the man, to ask for explanations, to express concern and resentment, with the consequence of making the man move further away; the latter will feel even more oppression and will need even more time to get out of his stress status.

In these cases, the advice I can give women is to leave the man alone for a few hours or a few days; after solving his problem, he will return to be more affectionate than before, also considering that his need for solitude has been respected.

Another advice I feel like giving to women is not to depend totally on men and their emotional state: cultivate various hobbies and interests, go out periodically with friends; in this way the periods of separation from the partner will be less hard and the rapprochement more joyful.

Also women face cyclical periods of stress: in those moments they are taken by pessimism and have negative feelings both towards their partner and towards the entire world. Even in times when their bond is going well and they feel that they have all the love in the world inside them, they suddenly end up having days of emotional stress.

In those cases, they do not dwell on a single problem, big or small: they are in a state of confusion and perceive past, future or just potential problems; sometimes, they raise problems for which there is no solution.

Unlike men, in these negative cycles, women do not lock themselves up in mutism, but have an enormous need to be listened to, reassured, and understood.

In these cases, I advise men to listen carefully to their spouses, to indulge them, not to oppose them, even if they expose you to absurd problems: it is time to support your partners, to try to entertain them, to give them hugs and love.

In this way, they will come out of their state of stress happier than before, they will show their gratitude in a thousand ways and your relationship will be positively affected.

Handling fights

Just as dialogue is essential for the strengthening of the couple's relationship, so arguments are destructive for the couple itself. If a couple started to quarrel every day, the feelings of love would progressively decrease until they disappear completely, and this would lead to the end of the relationship.

Which is obvious: you decide to be with another person because you are happier in two. The moment you live with fights and stress you are led to think that you were better off alone or that the one you are with is not the right person.

The most frequent reasons that lead to a quarrel are the following: money, education of children, mutual responsibilities, spare time. However, these are only apparent reasons for an argument, in reality you fight because you do not feel loved.

If a spouse does not feel loved, they will have negative feelings inside of them and instead of expressing their desire for love, they will tend to accuse the partner of something, triggering a quarrel.

If, for instance, a woman has been worried about her husband who came home late, she will tend to express herself with phrases like this: "How could you be so late! What should I think of you!" The husband, for his part, does not perceive that his wife has been worried about him and will tend to justify himself brusquely, claiming technical reasons such as traffic, or will minimize by saying that one cannot be as punctual as clockwork.

The message his wife will perceive is this: the delay is justified and what he was doing was certainly more important than their relationship. At this point it is obvious that we are getting into an argument.

Many times, the technical reason for the quarrel is not so important; how something is said is much more important than what it is said. Language is only a small part of communication: the tone of voice, the gestures, the gaze are important.

The same words can be said in a sweet and loving tone or in an aggressive tone. Depending on these two ways of expressing themselves, the same discussion can lead to an embrace or a destructive argument.

Men and women, having different sensibilities, quarrel and suffer from quarrels for different reasons.

A woman usually argues because her feelings are belittled: the man is inclined to play down by saying that everything is fine, that the woman's concern is excessive, offers practical solutions to the problem.

As a result, the woman does not feel listened to. The woman needs to feel understood and loved: for her feelings come before reason. And this should always be considered by men in order to avoid quarrels.

A man, on the other hand, usually quarrels because he senses the woman's disapproval. In the above example, the man will not feel the woman's concern, resulting from his delay: he will feel attacked, blamed and will get defensive, sometimes even uttering crude words; actually, the circumstance of not getting the woman's approval makes him suffer.

A man tends to deal with quarrels, generally, through two attitudes. Sometimes he attacks verbally, intimidating the woman. This attitude will eventually intimidate the woman, who will close in on herself and the relationship will fall apart, as the initial attraction will cease altogether.

Other times the man voluntarily decides to avoid quarrels by breaking off the dialogue and avoiding confrontation. It is clear, even in this case, that, with time, the couple's relationship will weaken.

The woman, on the other hand, tends to resolve systematic quarrels either by trying to pretend that everything is fine or by taking the blame for all the arguments of the couple. It goes without saying that this is also a wrong attitude: in this case, over time, the woman will be sucked into the vortex of resentment and the couple will collapse.

I recommend avoiding quarrels, but in the right way.

If you realize that a discussion is becoming a quarrel, it is a good idea to stop for a few hours to assess the matter from different points of view. Then it is essential to find an agreement: as with all problems, communication and dialogue are a panacea for resolving them.

You must not avoid problems and misunderstandings; you must avoid destructive arguments.

Therefore, it is necessary to communicate sincerely, tactfully expressing negative feelings as well. You have to learn to know each other more and more using the right words and tones in every situation, taking into account your partner's feelings and trying not to make them suffer.

In the example above, a good way to avoid a fight is as follows.

When the husband is late, the woman could say, "I was worried about you. Next time I'd like you to give me a heads-up in case you're late; I'd feel better."

The husband, for his part, could apologize for making his wife worry, paying attention to everything she says, without replying in a negative way.

In an advanced stage of a happy couple's relationship, one could also practice asking the other person, "What would you do in this negative situation? What words should I use to make you less angry or worried?"

For a happy and lasting relationship, dialogue, negotiation, sincerity, and transparency are essential qualities to be cultivated day by day.

Communicating a negative state of mind

We have said that there is a remedy for all problems in a couple: you have to communicate, negotiate, and approach each other with love.

We also said that the best way to avoid a quarrel is to move away from the problem, take a few hours to reflect and then communicate when the mood is more serene.

But if you feel betrayed, if you want to communicate a negative feeling, what is the best way to approach your partner?

What to communicate is important, but communicating it correctly, so as not to provoke the other person's anger and an argument, is even more important.

Before communicating a negative feeling, you should reflect individually on your feelings and structure a speech to your partner. You should first express your anger, sadness, and fears, then your sorrow and love.

Here is an example of how to correctly communicate a negative feeling.

Let's imagine that it is a couple's wedding anniversary and the wife has planned a romantic date, has prepared for the evening wearing a sexy dress and is looking forward to her husband coming home.

The husband comes home and candidly asks: "Why are you wearing such a beautiful dress?".

The wife, disappointed, lingers for a while until she is certain that the husband has forgotten about the anniversary and replies: "Today is our anniversary!".

The correct way to handle this situation, on the wife's side, without provoking an argument, is to retire to the bedroom for a few minutes and reflect on how to communicate the disappointment.

You need to fix in your mind all the elements of the speech you want to deal with or it would even be appropriate to write a note.

The content of this speech could be like this: "Darling, I am angry that you have forgotten about our wedding anniversary. It saddens me that you have not remembered such an important event. I'm afraid I'm not the center of your thoughts. I've been preparing for you since this morning. In any case, I'm sorry, perhaps I'm too demanding; perhaps I've been unlovely lately.

I love you and I forgive you for not remembering our anniversary. I know how much you work for the family, and these things can happen. I'm happy to be with you. Thank you for everything you do for us every day. I feel like the happiest woman in the world and now I want to celebrate with you with a romantic dinner. Honey, shall we treat ourselves to a few hours of magic?"

What man would not hug his woman after she gave him such beautiful emotions?

That is how an evening that could result in a bad fight, can, by communicating your feelings in a sincere and correct way, become one of the most beautiful of your life.

You should not hide your true emotions, even if negative, otherwise they will, sooner or later, turn into resentments.

In this regard, here is how men mistakenly tend to hide their feelings: they can resort to anger when they are afraid of not being loved; they can resort to presumption if they do not feel worthy of something; they can shut themselves away in silence to escape pain.

Likewise, here is how women could conceal their true feelings: they can resort to anxiety to hide their disappointments and sadness; they can resort to hope to escape suffering; they can resort to love to fill their frustrations and dissatisfactions.

You should avoid hiding your true feelings not only towards your partner, but above all towards yourself.

Stopping to reflect periodically for a few hours, before communicating negative feelings, is not only good for the couple, but above all for oneself.

Reflecting on negative feelings also helps to overcome old traumas of the past, which emerge in us periodically, conditioning our present and our future.

Stopping to analyze our negative moods helps us to grow, to develop our capacity for analysis and to become better women or men: it is a useful exercise, first, to love ourselves.

Managing crisis situations

As we have seen in previous chapters, sooner or later, for any couple there will be the period of crisis.

The important thing is to know how to face it in the right way.

If you are reading this guide and if you want to put its contents into practice, you will surely face the moments of crisis based on a solid relationship focused on love and harmony.

However, in the pathological phase of the relationship, there are some elements that you need to focus on more, which can help you overcome the various difficulties and fights.

First, you need to understand the partner's reasons before acting or reacting to a certain behavior. You should not limit yourself to appearances before judging, but you should be willing to know the background, the way your partner was raised, the environment in which his or her personality developed.

We all carry within us the traumas and wounds of the past, some more clearly, others less so. Knowing everyone's history helps you understand certain behaviors that you would not understand if you stopped at appearances. Being sensitive to your partner's past can avoid many arguments and improve the relationship.

Secondly, you need to manage time well. Time is the most important resource we have: we can sell it to someone (e.g. the employer), but we cannot buy it. When faced with important decisions to make, especially about the couple's life, we need to spend the right amount of time.

It is also necessary to devote the necessary time to the couple's relationship to cultivate and nurture it with love and devotion. Both the amount of time you devote and the quality are important.

Especially if you're going through a crisis, devote less to work and more to your relationship. Don't relate to your partner only when you are tired from work and can't wait to sleep.

Don't live life in a monotonous, predictable or conflictual way. Set yourself small positive goals every day in order to live a happy relationship: make small gifts, small surprises that your partner does not expect. And don't go to bed unless you are sure that you have given your partner at least a little bit of joy during the day. Make every day special: build your couple's love nest every day.

Always offer your support and emotional outreach: behave with the other person the way you would like them to behave with you; apply the golden rule in the relationship as well.

Also, do not oppress the other person with restrictions, jealousies, prohibitions. The couple is not a prison: everyone must feel free, have their own spaces of autonomy and cultivate their passions. This is the only way the partner will feel free to be authentic and spontaneous with you. Always remember: nobody forces you to sleep in the same bed. Your law must be that of love.

Moreover, in times of crisis, it is even more necessary to be willing to accept differences in character, without wanting to change the partner. Every issue must be resolved through compromise and dialogue: giving something to the other's reasons avoids many quarrels and misunderstandings.

Another golden rule is to listen with interest and curiosity to the other person, without taking a critical attitude and without judging. Some people don't even listen to their partner's words and are ready to contradict them right away. Sometimes silence is golden and the partner is not looking for advice, they just want to be listened to and understood to feel better.

Finally, another way to improve your damaged relationship is to limit your reactions to the current situation you are facing, without bringing up similar circumstances or even unresolved different situations that happened in the past.

Many couples tend to throw things at each other that no longer have anything to do with the current situation, with the only consequence that a small problem can take on disproportionate dimensions.

Coping with infidelity

Your partner cheated on you? Do you feel like the world's falling apart on you and you feel like a loser?

I know how it feels because I have been in this situation several times.

First, I want to tell you that this situation is common to millions of people: statistics say that almost 50% of couples will find themselves in a similar situation.

Secondly, you need to analyze the reasons that led to this: have you neglected your partner? Have you had disagreements about fundamental values in life or irreconcilable character incompatibilities? Is it only the partner's fault, who tends to cheat?

There can be many reasons behind infidelity.

What matters now, after reflecting on the reasons for infidelity, is how do you want to deal with adultery: do you want to forgive, or should you acknowledge that that person is not for you?

The final decision will be up to you alone, because only you know how much you love that person, what your family situations are, what you can tolerate and what you cannot.

If you are only engaged, for instance, you may decide with fewer constraints how to behave; if you are married with children, your decision will also affect other people's lives.

My opinion, in general, is that if a person has cheated on us, it is useless to continue: the magic and trust has broken and it is difficult, albeit not impossible, to start again.

However, I do not judge; as a fiancé I forgave several times, even though I was aware that the story was over.

When it comes to feelings, one should not judge. Sometimes the human mind is weak.

An incident that made me think was my barber who committed suicide after being left by his girlfriend. A few days earlier he had asked an acquaintance of mine: "What do you think about those who commit suicide after being left?" And my acquaintance answered lightly: "They're stupid."

Sometimes, during a relationship, a partner completely and naively relies on a person who is not worthy of them, putting everything aside; friends, personal interests, sometimes even family.

In these cases, the eventual breakup has a devastating effect on the psyche of the person who has been cheated.

Therefore, I do not judge those who want to forgive and the purpose of this guide is also to give suggestions on how to rebuild the relationship.

If you have strong character, if you understand that that person is not for you, if that person makes you deny your basic principles, it is better to break up.

If, for instance, you are a fervent Catholic and a partner had cheated on you on the grounds that you are too traditionalist and do not share the practice of couple swapping, being condescending to them could be even more devastating in the long term than the separation.

However, if you have the will and the strength to leave or accept the breakup of the relationship after the infidelity, it is a good thing: it means that you know you deserve more; that you can find better and that person was not for you.

If you love that person madly and hope to salvage the relationship, I am telling you that's possible too. Surely it is difficult, because it takes a long period of reconstruction of the relationship to renew the initial trust and feelings of love and tranquility.

I know some couples who are happy after overcoming marital infidelity. The commitment to rebuild trust can certainly lead to strengthen the couple and live a happy love relationship.

I remember a while ago I went to a faith meeting held by Claudia Koll. I was so impressed by her faith and dedication to others that I find it absurd that she has participated in erotic films in the past.

If I had not seen these films with my own eyes, I wouldn't have believed it. This is just one of many examples of how a person can also change for the better.

Back to us, though, how to rebuild the couple, or at least not to lose that person if you are not ready? Let us make some general assumptions that apply to all couples.

Never be jealous and possessive. Even if you are, practice smoothing out this flaw. Think about it: what does jealousy bring? Certainly, unnecessary fights, and fights have a long-term effect on feelings, as we have seen in previous chapters.

Those who feel oppressed by their partner will repress a desire for freedom that could lead to the breakup of the relationship or infidelity. So, paradoxically, if you are obsessively jealous you might get a different result from what you wanted, your partner might look for another person who is more joyful, less quarrelsome and who makes them feel freer in general. Jealousy is a feeling that is natural in us, yet stupid at the same time, because it certainly does not bring any benefit within the couple.

Therefore, it is important to practice not to show possessiveness or jealousy. On the contrary, you have to be attractive: have a thousand interests, not depend on your partner, feel confident, entertain your partner and discover new things together.

What to do if you suspect that a woman or a man is cheating on you?

Same rule applies as above: first, keep calm and do not let yourself be carried away by anger and jealousy. If you get carried away with negative feelings, you will lose points and the relationship will suffer. Think that your rival wants nothing more than to take you down, making you seem jealous, possessive, and nervous in general.

So, what to do? If you are not particularly committed to your partner, if you are willing to break your bond in case, they cheat on you, look into it: the cheater always makes even coarse missteps. Not everyone is willing to tolerate infidelity and it is right to break it off and then look for a more honest and sincere person.

But what if you love your partner and you do not want to lose them for any reason in the world?

Act as if nothing happened: do not investigate and do not try to catch your partner in the act. If you catch your partner in the act of cheating on you, you will suffer whilst the two lovers will be joined more in their guilt.

Unfortunately, there is the fascination of the forbidden: people like what is nasty and if what they like also causes suffering in a person, the pleasure is multiplied.

Therefore, do not try to track down your partner at the location of the prohibited meeting; do not check their mobile phone and do not argue out of jealousy.

If you argue with your partner because of another man or woman, you will only be entertaining them during their amorous encounter. I have often witnessed couples of lovers laughing at their jealous husband or wife because of several episodes. There are women or men who, when their jealous partner calls, even have sex with their lover, for a pure erotic game.

These things may sound absurd, but I assure you that they are real things and reality often exceeds imagination. The human soul is complex and interpreting it comprehensively is a chimera.

So, if you want to keep your relationship, ignore the rival completely. Even if they' re a mutual acquaintance, don't mention their name. If the cheating partner asks you for an opinion about that person, you speak well, saying that they are nice people. If you say that they are a smart, dangerous, mysterious person who is hiding something, you will only increase your rival's points.

Well, if you think about it, it's something normal. When a parent wants to give advice to their kid about their ideal partner, they usually get the opposite effect. Love is a partly irrational feeling and what is not ideal often attracts the most.

Therefore, tolerate the rival: if you use the right techniques, you will be the winner.

If you want to win against your rival, improve yourself and your relationship: become an interesting, fun, confident person. Be affectionate, but at the same time make it clear that without that person you would have a thousand other opportunities. Take the advice I gave you in previous chapters.

Remember, you are in a position of advantage over your partner. You have an established relationship that is growing day by day. The partner may be experiencing the moment of initial passion, but then everything will end and the first differences in character will begin. If your bond is strong, sooner or later your rival will succumb, and you will stay with the woman or man you love.

What do you do if your partner confesses to cheating on you and asks you for forgiveness?

As I wrote above, you must follow your heart. If you love that person, why not give them another chance? *Errare humanum est* and it could happen to anyone. Of course, it is necessary to rebuild the relationship, the trust that has been broken, but nothing is impossible: I know couples who have overcome this situation and are closer together than ever.

If you decide to salvage the relationship, however, you must take care not to constantly throw their mistake in the other person's face. You must never ask the details of the infidelity: it is better not to know than to continue to suffer for the past. If you touch the old wounds, they will never heal.

If you live the present always looking to the past your relationship will wear out, you will sever the bond and suffer twice.

So, it is important to create a new beginning with the person you love. You have decided to forgive, and the past no longer exists; besides, you cannot change the past. So, let's leave our skeletons in the closet!

What to do instead if the partner confesses the infidelity, does not want to end the story with you, but feels undecided on what to do?

In this case there are two different situations to deal with. The first case is when your partner asks you for a period of reflection. In this circumstance it is obvious that the outcome of this period will be negative.

The reflection period is nothing more than an excuse to gain time and have two people at your feet. In this case, you are the first to break it off: play it early and follow all the strategies I will explain in the next chapter.

If, on the other hand, the person you love, after confessing the infidelity, tells you that they have had, and still have, a period of sentimental disbandment, but does not ask you for any pause for reflection, in that case, if you love that person so much, forgive and move on.

In this case, it is likely your partner will cheat on you again. Avoid intercepting encounters with your rival, do not show jealousy; allow your partner to date the other person as well. If you fight because of the other person, you will play into the other person's hands.

If you really love your partner, it is wiser to share them and play even. Love is a militia and, with the right techniques, as I explained above, you will win against any rival. It will then be up to you to decide if it is worth continuing with the person you love or not. But you must decide as the winner, at your own pace and according to your wishes.

An example of managing infidelity: Angelica and I

To better explain the above concepts, I will tell you a story, which lasted several years, lived directly by me. Obviously, I will omit my ex-girlfriend's real name and some irrelevant details, for privacy reasons.

Those were my years at university. I had been engaged for a few years to Angelica, a brunette girl, pretty, attractive, and intelligent, whom I loved very much. The story between us was going well, in my opinion: when we went out, we had fun, we had common interests, we never quarreled and we exchanged promises of eternal love.

I had always treated her well and I was highly respected, both by her and her family.

One night, with nothing to presage, she told me she had to talk to me. I knew something was wrong, and I exclaimed, "Tell me!"

She looked away from my eyes and said to me, "I have to confess something bad I did. I kissed another guy. He took me by surprise, and I gave in.”

Overwhelmed, with my heart pounding, I replied: “But did he use violence?”

“No,” said Angelica, “I let myself be tempted and didn’t reject him. I am mortified. I ask your forgiveness because I love you and I want to continue to be with you.”

I, who for a moment had thought it was all over between us, hugged her and said, forcing myself to smile: “I forgive you, but don’t ever do it again. I love you!” We exchanged new promises of love and then decided to dine at a pizzeria talking about other more pleasant things. Of course, I did not ask for the details of the cheating. It would only lead to a fight.

I will not hide it, my dear readers, that when I returned home, I felt the world fall on me. I had read books about seduction and relationships for years and I knew very well that when a woman cheats, there is hardly a lack of involvement, the emotional and sentimental aspect with her lover. And then, was I sure it was just one kiss between them?

What could I have done? Leave her? My inner answer was, "Absolutely not. I love her too much and I can only see my future next to her." So, I decided to continue despite being aware that I had a rival. I convinced myself that maybe I would be able to recover the relationship and that the kiss was a mistake without consequences. In fact, I already doubted that Angelica would ever cheat on me again.

For the following two months, neither of us mentioned the problem that had arisen, and we continued our relationship. I tried to be even sweeter, more romantic, and reliable than I used to be. I did not show jealousy and tried to avoid fights altogether. I tried to make her have fun and prove my love every day.

Actually, I secretly managed to gather information about my rival from mutual friends. He was a cute and funny guy, but as a person, he was worth a lot less than me.

However, he had conquered Angelica's heart, and I had to fight with all the weapons at my disposal.

First, I knew I had the advantage, because she had "chosen" me for years.

I had the impression that she was cheating on me: sometimes she had her head in the clouds; sometimes the buses made "strange" delays; other times she received phone calls that she interrupted without answering. They were clear symptoms of a new infidelity.

One day I followed her without being caught and my suspicions became certain: I saw her with him laughing, joking, and kissing.

Again, I decided not to face the situation and to continue as if nothing had happened. I was not ready to lose the person I loved, with whom I had built all the dreams of my future.

One night came the dreaded yet expected moment.

Angelica said to me: "I should have told you long ago that I'm seeing someone else. I love you and I do not want to lose you, that's why I didn't tell you until now. It is only fair, though, that you know it. I'm struggling because I think I have feelings for the other person too." That said, she burst into tears.

We hugged and remained silent for a few minutes.

Then I replied: "For what you told me it would probably be normal to react badly. But I feel I still love you and I am not ready to lose you. I have a deal to offer you, to suffer as little as possible."

She looked at me doubtful and asked, "What kind of deal?"

Looking away from her eyes I replied, "I propose that we continue to see each other twice a week, doing the same things as always. You can continue to see whoever you want and understand what you feel. I, too, will devote myself more to friends and other interests. I think this is the best way not to suffer."

Surprised by this speech Angelica replied: "Are you sure that's enough for you? Maybe it's not right."

To this objection I replied: "I love you and with this solution I will hardly notice what is happening. So, I'm sure."

After giving it a minute's thought, she said, "Okay, it's a deal! If it is okay with you, I'm more comfortable too."

As I predicted, the agreement did not have a great backlash on our relationship, also because I, as usual, did not show jealousy and tried to make the most of the moments we spent together. Even in the intimacy it seemed to me that nothing had changed.

In the meantime, I enrolled in the gym, I started a theater class, I went out more with old friends. I also took great care of my look and read books about seduction.

However, deep down inside, on the one hand, I was jealous and, on the other, I was beginning to wonder if it was worth continuing.

One evening, after moments of intimacy, she said to me, "Sometimes I feel guilty towards the other person. He suffers that I'm seeing you."

At that point, I replied angrily: "But when he was seeing you during our engagement, I don't suppose he ever worried about me? In fact, I imagine him even laughing at me for not noticing anything."

Reflecting for a moment, and smiling faintly, she replied: "Forget what I said: mine was just a passing mood."

What had happened was quite alarming: her feelings for the other person were increasing. Words were useless and I had to find a strategy not to lose Angelica.

The next evening, while going out with my friend Antonio on the waterfront in Salerno, I had the opportunity I was looking for. My friend pointed out to me a beautiful blonde girl who was looking at me and urged me to go and meet her. She immediately greeted me with a smile and all I had to do was introduce myself to her to make a funny and seductive speech.

The next night I went out with this new girl making sure I was seen in a very crowded place, where, in theory, Angelica could have seen me too.

Instead, Angelica's sister saw me, and at that moment, I deliberately took the pretty blonde girl by the hand. I had no doubt that Angelica would be warned; this gave me enormous satisfaction.

Angelica's reaction was worse than I expected. As soon as she saw me, almost screaming, she said: "You didn't waste time replacing me! Do you like the little blonde? Did you kiss her?"

Maliciously smiling, I replied: "Angelica, calm down! Do you even realize that you are having an affair with another guy and I've never made a jealous scene? Aren't I free to date someone else, too?"

With eyes flashing with anger she exclaimed: "But the one you're seeing is a whore! And then it is no longer true that I'm seeing someone else. Just this afternoon I broke up with him. I made him cry a lot because I told him that the only one I love is you."

"So what?" I replied with a certain satisfaction.

"And so now we can get back together. I now know who I love. But you must never see the blonde girl again," she said outragedly.

Trying to hide a smile, I replied, "Give me a day to think about it. A lot has happened in these past few months and I want to think about it!"

Despite Angelica's cries and wails, I did not tell her my positive decision until the next day.

Dear readers, what do you say, did she deserve a little punishment? I felt like she did.

Our renewed engagement lasted just over a month. One night she told me that she had cheated on me again. I was expecting it, and I offered the old deal again. She accepted and we continued to see each other for a few months, as before.

Meanwhile, however, my feelings towards Angelica were diminishing and, above all, I was now confident that we could not have a future. I went on with her only out of habit, out of inertia.

Then came the moment when I fell in love with another girl, named Fiorella, pretty, sweet, and serious.

So, I told Angelica that I did not want to see her anymore, because I had gotten engaged to Fiorella.

Angelica, desperate, said to me, "Please don't do this to me. I swear to you, I left him. I love you!" But I was adamant in my decision.

Then she went on to say, "At least let's continue with our agreement. When you suffered for me, I was always there. Now you want to leave me completely!"

To which I replied: "You were the one who cheated on me after four years. And your man also contributed to our breakup. He did not deserve any respect! Who deserves respect is Fiorella, who is unaware of all our complicated relationships. I am sorry, what I can offer you now is only friendship. And I am not interested in us going out alone anymore. Now I have a girlfriend!"

Angelica, like so many of my ex-girlfriends, would call me back several times to get back together. But that is another story and we will have to tell it another time.

Winning back your ex-partner

Breaking up a relationship is always a negative, sometimes dramatic moment, especially for those who are being left.

This chapter is specifically dedicated to those who find themselves in this situation and feel lost, useless, unhappy, and without a perspective.

I know this situation because I have been through it several times.

The good thing is that with the right techniques, 90% of the relationships can be salvaged. Moreover, the longer the relationship has lasted, the greater the likelihood of recovery.

Dear reader, if you find yourself in the situation described above, do not get down and follow what I'm about to tell you. With my personal experience and my studies on the psychology of the couple, you will be able to win back your loved one.

The first rule you must follow if you have just been left is not to call the ex: ignore them completely, don't call them and don't meet them. Storming them with phone calls or go begging them to take you back will have the opposite effect. Who likes someone who goes begging for love? This behavior is the antithesis of seduction. If you do this your ex-partner will be even more convinced of the decision made and the hopes of winning them back will be reduced to zero.

You therefore need a period of reflection to understand the reasons for the break-up and whether it is worth salvaging. As I wrote above, if the causes of the rupture stem from disagreements over life's values, it may not be worth it. However, you are the author of your life and you are free to want to salvage the relationship anyway.

The second fundamental step to recover the relationship, but also to feel better in general, is to rebuild self-esteem and spiritual well-being, which have been diminished by abandonment.

To do this, it is necessary to create or recreate social relationships and dedicate oneself to new interests.

Even during a couple's relationship, one should not neglect friends and social relationships. However, if you have not done so, it is time to devote more time to old friendships and above all it is time to go out.

I know, the first days after breaking up you are not in the mood to go out, and perhaps even crying or listening to sad songs can help relieve the tension.

However, it is essential to get organized and go out soon to engage in pleasant things such as dancing, movies, pubs and restaurants, out-of-town trips.

Then, you need to create new interests, also with the aim of meeting new people. New hobbies are essential. There are hundreds of things that can make you happier: travelling, doing theatre, joining a cultural association. If you don't already do it, you should join a gym, which can also improve your physical appearance.

You must overcome your limits. If you like to dance, but you are shy, you must overcome this limit. If you want to travel, do not wait to be rich to do it. Do not put off opportunities to be happy.

Meet new people, even strangers. Show yourself cheerful and playful and smile at everyone. For the principle of reciprocity, you will see that your friends and your social sphere of influence will increase.

In a few weeks you will feel better and have already made new friends.

Take advantage now to post on social networks some photos of you in good company.

While in the days following the breakup, it is not advisable to publish anything, when you have recovered it is appropriate, without exaggeration, to publish photos in which you appear serene. But why all this?

As I was saying above, in the first few weeks after the breakup, your ex-partner must not hear from you. They must wonder what happened to you.

Later, they will see, for instance on Facebook, some photos where you radiate serenity and they will realize that your life does not depend on theirs. You will begin to trigger in them the mechanisms of curiosity and jealousy, which will then lead to winning back your partner.

It is not appropriate, at this moment, to post photos with other women or other men: it could be interpreted by the former partner as something to make him or her jealous. So, at this time, be moderate on socials.

But how long do you have to ignore the ex? Extensive psychology studies suggest trying a first contact after a month. In my experience, three weeks would be good.

What to do if in the meantime you have not heard from your partner and how to make the first contact?

The most suitable and discreet means is a text message or similar because it allows an indirect approach and gives more time to refine the reconquest strategy.

Instead of drawing up an academic list on how to act to win back your partner, at this stage, I would rather tell you two stories of reconquest that I experienced directly.

How I won Lara back

Several years ago, after almost a year of engagement, Lara left me on the phone. Sure, we lived several miles apart, but being left over the phone is not nice. So, following my protest, I got to see her in person to better understand the reasons for the breakup.

I loved Lara very much, but on reflection, I thought I had submitted too much in "begging" for a meeting. That is why I called back and told her that there was no longer any need for the meeting. She was not expecting it and told me that the causes of the breakup were that I was too traditionalist and stiff. At that point, feeling offended, I told her to find someone else and hung up.

At that point, after a few hours, Lara's cousin, Sara, called me and said: "Francesco, Lara gives you the opportunity to see her and you don't go to the appointment!". To those words I replied: "But she's already decided: it's useless!" To which Sara exclaimed: "So it's true that you're stiff!"

With Sara, who was married and much older than us, I had a special relationship: I confided in her and often went to her house, as we lived nearby.

The first days after the breakup were terrible for me: I cried and listened to the saddest songs by Marco Masini and Gatto Panceri. I desperately wanted to call Lara, but I knew I was neither in the right mood nor was it the right strategy.

I had to do something and decided to change my look: I went to the men's hairdresser and had my hair curled. I bought me some trendy clothes, enrolled in judo, and started going out again.

With my friend Antonio we started randomly stopping all the girls we met on the waterfront in Salerno and this made me feel good: I was able to meet new girls and improve my self-esteem. It is always gratifying when you arouse interest in a woman.

I did not publish anything about me on social networks so both Lara and Sara did not have any more news about me.

I could not forget Lara and the pain for her loss, despite my distractions, increased. I had to do something.

After three weeks of silence, I decided to send a strategic text message.

This is what I wrote to her: "Hello Lara. I have thought a lot about your words, and I agree with you that I have too stiff a character. I therefore agree with your decision to break up. I spent the best moments of my life with you. I will miss you. Francesco."

Needless to say, after that message, I was on my cell phone every second checking for an answer. I tortured myself thinking maybe I'd written a stupid text. Why write those things when I wanted to say, "I'm dying without you"?

Fortunately for me, the wait wasn't too long. After a couple of hours my cell phone vibrated and when I saw Lara's name my heart began to beat like crazy.

She wrote me: "I'm surprised by your words, but at the same time I'm glad that you recognized your mistakes and agreed with my decision. I was sad a few days and wondered how you are. Sometimes I reflect on the fact that our story could have had a different ending."

I was very pleased to receive her reply. It's not at all obvious for an ex-girlfriend to answer you.

I analyzed Lara's message in detail, which seemed contradictory to me. On the one hand she was happy that I accepted her decision; on the other hand she reflected on several possible epilogues of our story. In any case, she asked me how I was doing and I had to answer.

I decided not to answer right away, so as not to appear submissive.

The next day I wrote to her: "I was sad a few days too, but now I'm fine and I'm going out almost every night. Thank you for your answer. We'll catch up."

I never heard from Lara again for that day.

The next day, however, her cousin Sara called me. She asked me how I was and if I wanted to go see a movie at her place. I pretended to be undecided, but then I said yes. I was really looking forward to such an opportunity! Sara was very close to Lara and, at the very least, it would be a chance to get information about my beloved.

I prepared meticulously for the appointment: I wore fashionable clothes, a refined perfume, I fixed my hair with gel and foam.

As soon as I got to Sara's house, I had an apparition and my heart started pounding. Lara was there.

We greeted each other with a handshake, and I exclaimed: "Lara, you are here too!'?'"

"Sure, I'm staying at my cousin's and I like movies too. What happened to your hair?" She asked.

"I decided to change my look. Some people appreciate it," I replied in a mischievous tone.

"Well, that's what they all say," she said in an almost defiant tone. "How are you and what are you doing anyway?" She continued.

"I've joined the gym, I'm going out with friends and got a job," I smiled.

"I can't believe it. What kind of work?" She investigated.

"I'm being a playboy. I am taking a course in both theory and practice. Sure, I'm still a beginner, but I'm not doing badly," I said allusively.

"I wouldn't believe it even if I saw it with my own eyes! You?" She exclaimed amused.

"Well, in life everything changes. Then I certainly chose a sweet art," I said amused.

The conversation went on in this playful manner throughout the evening and I took care not to mention anything about our breakup.

We all sat down on the couch and started watching a movie. Sara asked what kind of movie we wanted to see: I voted for a horror movie, Lara for a romantic comedy. Of course, Sara pleases her cousin.

During the movie I almost had the feeling that Lara was touching my leg. In any case, I tried to avoid any physical contact with her. I wanted her to miss my skin. I even came up with a staging to help my cause.

I sent a text message to my friend Antonio saying, "I need an urgent favor. Have your friend Federica call me and ask me in a sensual voice when we meet. I'm with Lara and I'd like to make her jealous."

After about half an hour, during a love scene in the movie, I got a phone call. I answered and a female voice asked me: "Francesco, when will we see each other? Can you come to the usual bar afterwards?" I answered in a serious tone: "I'm at the movies now, I'll call you later or tomorrow. Have a nice evening!"

I took care to put the speakerphone on for a second. In any case, the female voice was clearly audible to the two cousins.

Lara did not say anything, but you could see her eyes were upset. I almost had the impression they were flickering. However, I did not linger looking her in the eyes, to avoid betraying myself: I had to be serious and avoid laughing at all costs.

At the end of the night, I had to figure out a strategic way to end the conversation.

When she greeted me, making it clear she

would kiss me on the cheek, I just gave her my hand. And when she said, "See you at the next casual movie!" I said, "Sure, in a year or two!"

I had a feeling the night had gone better than I expected. But I didn't have to go overboard in optimism: I had to continue my work of reconquest.

I decided to post a photo on Facebook where I was embraced by a beautiful friend of mine. We both smiled and, even though she was actually engaged and really just a friend of mine, the photo could look ambiguous. Then, from my experience, I knew that a jealous woman sees rivals even in the most innocent photos.

The next day there was absolute silence. She did not make herself heard and I began to think I had gone too far in posting a photo with another girl on Facebook.

The following day, however, much to my surprise, came the turning point.

Lara sent me a text message saying: "Hi Francesco. I've been thinking about us and I realized I said some things I didn't mean. Am I still in time to ask to see you? Are you free tonight?"

I immediately thought in my mind that the miracle had happened: I was so happy!

I replied: "I'm not free, but I think I can make myself free. I'll let you know later what time and where I'll see you."

I planned it down to the smallest detail: I prepared a nice speech and wore a genuinely nice green jacket. I even had time to take my car to the car wash.

The village where Lara lived was 25 miles from Salerno, my town. I was a couple of miles from the place where I was meeting Lara when I saw a beautiful brunette girl hitchhiking: she had a pretty face, a perfect physique and she was wearing a very attractive miniskirt. I decided to give her a lift. After showing me where she was going, she asked me: "You're not local. What are you doing here?"

"I'm going to my fiancée's," I replied, noting a certain disappointment in her eyes.

Anyway, when she arrived at her destination, the pretty girl said, "By the way, you're really a handsome guy!".

She waited a few seconds in the car for my answer, but I just said, "Thank you!"

With hindsight, I thought maybe I could ask for her phone number. But at that moment I loved Lara too much, and it was only right.

The time came for me to meet Lara. I had never seen her so beautiful: she had prepared herself to perfection, she had a heavenly smile and her eyes were so in love that I lost the light of reason.

We hugged without saying anything and exchanged a kiss on the lips more eloquent than a thousand words.

Then I asked her jokingly, "So I'm stiff?"

"Very," she joked too. Then she exclaimed, "I love you!"

"I love you more," I answered her.

That evening I had written on a piece of paper

a series of things to tell her.

But in the end I said nothing. Our mouths were too busy drinking the magic of love.

How I won back Marta

Now I'm going to tell you another story lived directly by me.

Marta, after two years of engagement, had left me. The reason was that she didn't feel the same feelings as before and our relationship had become too monotonous. In order to get closer to her, I did everything I should not have done: I begged her to come back with me, I apologized for having neglected her, and I was storming her with messages on her mobile phone.

She blocked me on the social networks, sent me a text message begging me to leave her alone and even had her mother call me to tell me that I shouldn't bother her anymore.

I had to change my strategy: continuing in this way I risked not only losing her forever as a girlfriend, but also losing her salute.

I came to my senses and decided to act as the seduction psychologists advise.

For about three weeks I disappeared completely, and I didn't contact her at all. The only exchange of texts was with her friend Laura, who asked me how I was and what I was doing. Again, I gave a cold, courteous answer.

Then I sent Marta a text message in which I agreed to end our relationship, acknowledged my mistakes and admitted that I would miss her so much, because we had lived unforgettable moments.

The days passed and there was no answer.

So I had to find a different strategy. I had to meet her, but at the same time make it seem purely random. I had to find the right opportunity.

Meanwhile, by chance I saw a post on Facebook in which Laura, Marta's friend, said she was going crazy to prepare for the criminal procedure exam: she had already taken it several times, with a negative result. I had just graduated in law and I had got the top marks in that subject.

So I offered to help her, telling her that it was a subject I liked, that I would also use it for competitive exams and that I was happy to listen to her in order to get her to pass the exam. I worked hard to review the exam in depth: for a month I explained all the lessons of criminal procedure to her and I listened and listened to her carefully.

When she wanted to talk to me about my ex, I told her I'd rather not talk about it and that it was over.

One day I had an invitation to attend a birthday party from Viviana, a mutual friend: she told me that she cared about my presence, that I shouldn't let myself be influenced if Marta was present and that I could bring a friend with me. I told her that, even if I had another engagement, I would come to the party.

That afternoon, among other things, I went to listen to the lessons of criminal procedure at Laura's house, who told me that she would go to the party with Marta. I told her I still did not know if I was going to be there.

So, I thought about the strategy I had to follow to earn points with Marta.

I arrived at Viviana's party very late, when everyone was already dancing, but before the cake. Antonio, my seduction expert friend, was with me. We approached the birthday girl first, wishing her a happy birthday, and then we greeted Marta and Laura. I said to Laura: "Ah, instead of studying you indulge in nightly revelry. Tomorrow I'll fail you."

Laura jokingly replied: "Don't worry, I'll know how to make it up to you."

I just reached out to my ex-girlfriend Marta and said, "What's up?"

"Fine," she said, "it's a great party with good music."

"I'm glad," I said. "See you later!"

Antonio and I then walked away, quickly grabbed something to eat and drink and headed towards the dance floor.

There were several cheerful and cute girls: it was worth trying to approach them. Antonio knew my strategy and, after having probed the ground, we approached the two girls who looked at us more than the others and gave us positive signals by smiling in an inviting way.

All we had to do was say our name and we already started dancing with sexy movements. Antonio, as usual, also started to kiss her; instead, I was content to dance with the girl I had just met and to have fun. In the strategy I had devised, I could not go beyond that.

Occasionally, I'd have Antonio peek at what Marta and Laura were doing. He told me that several times he had caught them looking at us surprised.

Right after the cake time, I pretended they were calling me. We said a quick hello to the birthday girl and ran away. Needless to say, as we left, we didn't even look at Marta and Laura.

The next day, when Laura asked me for explanations for my coldness, I told her that I was not too pleased to see my ex, who, by the way, had not answered my last message. She also asked me if I was planning to go out with the girl I had met the night before and I told her, with a smile, that I was undecided.

After a few hours I got the following text message: "Hi, it's Marta. It was nice to see you again last night. I wanted to apologize because I didn't reply to your message last time. I thought I had answered, but I completely forgot."

I decided not to answer her right away. She, by the way, had made me wait long enough for her answer, too.

After two days, I replied:

"Don't worry, Marta. I had almost forgotten! Kisses. See you soon."

She immediately replied: "Obviously I agree to remain friends. Kisses to you too!"

I decided not to answer.

In the meantime, thanks also to my efforts, Laura passed the exam with a score of 27/30, an excellent grade. She thanked me by offering me dinner in a restaurant and asked me if I wanted to be paid. I replied in an almost offended tone, telling her that I had followed her out of friendship and I only did these things out of friendship.

We had a pleasant and carefree evening. After enjoying an excellent dessert Laura asked me if I had heard from her friend. I told her about the text message exchange and she, informing me that Marta had to take the civil law exam, asked me if I was willing to help her too. I pretended not to be so enthusiastic about it, but I told her that if she contacted me, I would accept.

As expected, after a few days, Marta sent me the following text message: "Hi. How are you? I'm having trouble with my civil law exam and I was wondering if you could help me."

Two hours later I replied: "All right, I accept under two conditions: the first is that we start immediately because time is tight and I must guarantee you a positive result of the exam; the second is that if you don't study, as you know, I will punish you."

You must know, dear reader, that I had already helped Laura in the past and, when she did not study enough, I pretended to punish her with a little slap during moments of intimacy. Each couple has its own characteristic language and, with this text message, I certainly evoked old emotions.

In any case, she accepted my conditions and the next day I was already at her house. The first few days I was quite cold and professional. I tried to avoid physical contact and direct allusions to our previous engagement.

Meanwhile I went out with large groups, posted photos on social networks, and surrounded myself with sweet friends.

Often, while I was with Marta, I got texts or phone calls from female friends I had to go out with at night. These circumstances, I noticed, annoyed Marta; but that was my purpose.

She would sometimes ask if it was just *friends* who contacted me, in allusive tones. I would minimize it by replying that they were friends, just met, of the group of Pino, a mutual friend of ours, who asked me for a ride in the car.

One night I saw Marta staring insistently at my neck.

"Why are you staring at me?" I asked her.

"Because you have lipstick on your neck. I see you didn't waste any time to replace me with another girl!" replied my ex.

She picked up a mirror and pointed out to me that it was just like she said.

It occurred to me that a few hours earlier I had been at breakfast with two very dear friends with whom there had never been anything, but, for fun, they kissed me and I kissed them, even on the lips.

I told Marta that it was all a joke, but she didn't seem to believe me. So I changed the subject and then we went back to our civil law lessons. Of course I could have pointed out to her that we were no longer engaged, that she had left me and I had every right to kiss whoever I wanted. However, it was not my aim to create a conflict. On the contrary, I was unintentionally arousing jealousy, and that might have helped me.

Besides, I remembered that when we got engaged, I was torn between her and an ex-girlfriend of mine who had gotten back in touch. She almost begged me to pick her. Everything was born out of feelings of jealousy and everything was coming together again with the same feelings, from Marta.

The next day my ex welcomed me dressed like a supermodel, with a fruity perfume and the short floral dress that I liked so much in the past.

She sat in front of me and asked me: "Swear to me that there isn't any other girl!"

Meanwhile, her legs touched mine and her hands touched me.

"I swear I love you!" I answered.

And we indulged in the sweetest kisses and hugs we had ever exchanged. And after hours and hours we were not satisfied. The passion was sky-high and we were closer than ever.

A few days later, however, in a moment of intimacy, I gave Marta a stronger slap. After leaving me she deserved it: but strangely enough, it was like a gift for her!

Conclusions

Dear reader, if you are in a couple's relationship, this manual offers you many ideas on how to improve or heal your relationship.

I have written this guide to help you live your relationship with greater enthusiasm, harmony and serenity.

Start from the assumption that you will never completely know your partner because each person has their secret soul, their uniqueness. This is not necessarily a bad thing, because there will always be new challenges, new things to discover so that you don't take anything for granted and don't fall into monotony.

As I said above, you have to be lovable if you want to be loved. We must try to avoid quarrels and try to resolve conflicts through mediation and compromise.

Then you have to take care of the emotional element: even if your relationship has lasted for several years, you have to be able to attract your loved one. In order to attract, you sometimes need to detach yourself: in general, what attracts is something far away, something that is considered precious.

Therefore, to arouse a touch of jealousy is sometimes healthy. Seduction is an art that should be cultivated not only in the initial moment of a relationship, but throughout the duration of the relationship. If you lull yourself on your laurels thinking that the relationship will last forever without caring for it, you risk compromising it forever.

I then dwelt in particular, also through my personal stories, on the strategies of reconquest of the partner who has severed a relationship.

With these strategies, if you don't make mistakes, in almost all cases, you will recover the relationship and find happiness. The longer the relationship has lasted, the closer the chances of recovery will be to one hundred percent.

We have examined two cases: the first, in which the dialogue, despite the breakup, has never completely broken. And we have seen that recovery strategies here are quite easy if you follow the techniques I teach.

We then analyzed the case where the partner broke all contact. In this case the recovery is slower and you have to start again from the friendship, after having succeeded, with the necessary strategies, to patch up the dialogue.

In both these situations it is necessary to use emotional and hypnotic techniques borrowed from psychology. You have to stimulate in your partner a substance called oxytocin, to push them straight into your arms.

As I explained above, to stimulate this substance, you need to act in three directions: to recall the memories and positive situations that allowed the partner to bond with you in the beginning; to mentally dominate the partner, through the principle of scarcity, making them understand that you have become a better person, successful and with many admirers; finally, you need to know how to sexually attract the partner with the right words and actions.

With these techniques the former partner will have no desire other than to return to your arms.

The purpose of this book is to provide guidance on how to improve or save your relationship and how to win back your former partner after the breakup of the relationship.

Remember, however, that a set of words, written in a book or guide, cannot change your life if the concepts described are not put into practice. Knowledge without action does not lead to results. Therefore, I invite you to reread this guide several times and put it into practice every day.

Dear reader, as you can imagine, word of mouth, sharing and comments are vital for an author. That is why I ask you, if you liked this guide, to write a review of my work.

If you have something to ask me in private, a specific case to submit and you want my advice you can contact me – besides my Facebook and Instagram profiles – at the following e-mail address: koatiyah@hotmail.it. I give you this little gift: my free advice.

If you want to deepen the topic of seduction, I suggest you also read my other guide: *Seducing women - The secrets of the seducer: The playboy techniques*. Here is the synopsis.

Seducing women is an art: how many girls are you missing because you don't know the right techniques?

In this eBook you will discover how to effectively pick up the best girls, with a delicious and magnetic seduction!

This guide is a comprehensive code of gallant strategies, aimed both at the shy and naive and at the malicious experimenters of erotic practices.

To seduce a woman, you do not have to appear romantic, friendly or a "good guy", but you need techniques, rules, artifices, experience.

Not all women are the same. You will require different techniques of seduction, depending on the concrete situation.

In this book, ample space will be dedicated to the techniques of approach in the most in the most diverse contexts: public places, holidays (both in Italy and abroad), universities, movie theaters, discos, chats.

We will reveal the mysteries to hypnotize every kind of woman with love: the naive, the shy, the experienced woman, the young girl, the mature woman or the engaged one.

After reading this guide, written by Francesco Cibelli, one of the most experienced Italian masters in the art of seduction, it will be within everyone's reach to conquer any woman, even the prettiest or most noble.

Moreover, at the end of the book, the author will reserve a pleasant surprise for the reader.

"I'm a young guy and I still don't know how to approach girls, but this eBook has helped me to pick up more girls in bars and clubs. Highly recommended for those seeking advice on seduction!"

Francesco Tesei

"I never had a problem getting girls but reading this guide I actually learned how to seduce in a magnetic and delicious way! Now I pick up girls even at the bus stop!"

Paolo Rieti

"My friends always talk to me about liquid love, and about how to talk to girls the right way so as to pick them up and seduce them. Well, in this book you will find a very up-to-date and interesting guide on how to have a magnetic and delicious seduction! Congratulations to the author."

Fabio Persico

"With this book seducing women seems a piece of cake, but is it true? I still have to try many of the techniques, but so far it seems to be better in picking up girls. So, kudos to the author."

Enzo Dellera